Churg-Strauss Syndrome

A Beginner's Quick Start Guide on Managing EGPA through Home Remedies and Diet, with Sample Recipes

mf

copyright © 2022 Patrick Marshwell

All rights reserved No part of this book may be reproduced, or stored in a retrieval system, or transmitted in any form or by any means, electronic, mechanical, photocopying, recording, or otherwise, without express written permission of the publisher.

Disclaimer

By reading this disclaimer, you are accepting the terms of the disclaimer in full. If you disagree with this disclaimer, please do not read the guide.

All of the content within this guide is provided for informational and educational purposes only, and should not be accepted as independent medical or other professional advice. The author is not a doctor, physician, nurse, mental health provider, or registered nutritionist/dietician. Therefore, using and reading this guide does not establish any form of a physician-patient relationship.

Always consult with a physician or another qualified health provider with any issues or questions you might have regarding any sort of medical condition. Do not ever disregard any qualified professional medical advice or delay seeking that advice because of anything you have read in this guide. The information in this guide is not intended to be any sort of medical advice and should not be used in lieu of any medical advice by a licensed and qualified medical professional.

The information in this guide has been compiled from a variety of known sources. However, the author cannot attest to or guarantee the accuracy of each source and thus should not be held liable for any errors or omissions.

You acknowledge that the publisher of this guide will not be held liable for any loss or damage of any kind incurred as a result of this guide or the reliance on any information provided within this guide. You acknowledge and agree that you assume all risk and responsibility for any action you undertake in response to the information in this guide.

Using this guide does not guarantee any particular result (e.g., weight loss or a cure). By reading this guide, you acknowledge that there are no guarantees to any specific outcome or results you can expect.

All product names, diet plans, or names used in this guide are for identification purposes only and are the property of their respective owners. The use of these names does not imply endorsement. All other trademarks cited herein are the property of their respective owners.

Where applicable, this guide is not intended to be a substitute for the original work of this diet plan and is, at most, a supplement to the original work for this diet plan and never a direct substitute. This guide is a personal expression of the facts of that diet plan.

Where applicable, persons shown in the cover images are stock photography models and the publisher has obtained the rights to use the images through license agreements with third-party stock image companies.

Table of Contents

Introduction	7
The Churg-Strauss Syndrome or "EGPA"	9
Symptoms of Churg-Strauss Syndrome (CSS)	12
Causes of Churg-Strauss Syndrome	16
Diagnosis	18
Diagnostic Criteria	21
Treatment of Churg-Strauss Syndrome	24
Lifestyle Changes to Manage Churg-Strauss Syndrome	25
The 3 Phases of CSS	30
Phase 1: Prodromal Phase	30
Phase 2: Eosinophilic Phase	32
Phase 3: Vasculitic Phase	35
Management Through Diet	39
A Balanced, Nutritious Diet	39
Limiting Unhealthy Fats	40
Managing Blood Sugar Levels	40
5-Step-by-Step Guide to Starting a Diet for Churg-Strauss Syndrome	42
Step 1: Consult with Your Healthcare Provider	42
Step 2: Educate Yourself on Anti-Inflammatory Foods	44
Step 3: Plan Balanced Meals	46
Step 4: Monitor and Adjust	49
Step 5: Stay Hydrated and Limit Processed Foods	53
Foods to Avoid	53
Foods to Eat	56
7-Day Meal Plan	58
Sample Recipes	61
Baked Spanish Mackerel Fillets	62
Udon Salmon Soup	63

Steamed Cauliflower and Curried Shrimp	65
Chia Seed and Strawberry Pudding	67
Low-Cholesterol Waldorf Salad	68
Quinoa-Based Oriental Salad	69
Broccoli Soup	70
Blueberry Flax Smoothie	71
Fried Eggs and Vegetables	72
Toasted Muesli	73
Lentil Stew	74
Salmon with Honey and Mustard	76
Cauliflower Pizza	77
Quinoa Stuffed Peppers	79
Tofu Scramble	81
Conclusion	**82**
FAQs	**85**
References and Helpful Links	**88**

Introduction

Churg-Strauss Syndrome (CSS), also known as Eosinophilic Granulomatosis with Polyangiitis (EGPA), is a rare form of blood vessel inflammation. It is characterized by the abnormal growth of white blood cells called eosinophils, which are normally present in small numbers and help fight infections. In individuals with CSS, eosinophils proliferate uncontrollably, causing damage to tissues and organs. The syndrome was first described by Drs. Churg and Strauss in 1951.

While there is no cure for CSS, various treatments are available to manage symptoms and prevent further damage. This guide will explore natural methods for managing CSS, focusing on diet and lifestyle remedies. Diet plays a crucial role in managing CSS, as certain foods can reduce inflammation while others may trigger flares. Identifying and avoiding trigger foods is essential for symptom management.

In addition to dietary changes, several natural methods such as supplements, herbs, and home remedies can help alleviate CSS symptoms. This beginner's quick-start guide will cover:

- What Churg-Strauss Syndrome is
- Its symptoms, diagnosis, and treatment options
- Lifestyle remedies
- The 3 Phases of CSS
- Management Through Diet
- 5-Step-by-Step Guide to Starting a Healthy Diet for Churg-Strauss Syndrome
- Foods to eat and avoid
- Sample recipes

Keep reading to learn more about CSS and discover various tips and techniques on how you can manage it naturally. We'll explore best practices, common pitfalls, and innovative solutions to help you master this essential web development skill.

The Churg-Strauss Syndrome or "EGPA"

Churg-Strauss syndrome (CSS), also known as eosinophilic granulomatosis with polyangiitis (EGPA), is a rare condition characterized by inflammation of the blood vessels, which can lead to damage in organs such as the lungs, heart, and brain. The condition was first described by Dr. Jakob Churg in 1951, with further contributions by Dr. Strauss in 1955. The reason for the name change from CSS to EGPA remains unclear.

The term "eosinophilic granulomatosis with polyangiitis" is derived from Greek: "eosinophilia" refers to an overabundance of eosinophils (a type of white blood cell), "granulomatosis" indicates the formation of small lumps in body tissue, and "polyangiitis" means inflammation of many blood vessels.

In CSS, inflammation occurs in blood vessels throughout the body, leading to potential organ damage. This condition is marked by an increased number of eosinophils, which are white blood cells that help fight infection. In CSS, eosinophils accumulate in various parts of the body, including the lungs, heart, and brain.

White blood cells, or leukocytes, are essential components of the immune system, protecting the body against infection and disease.

There are five types of white blood cells, each with a distinct function:

1. ***Neutrophils***: The most common type of white blood cell, neutrophils are the body's first line of defense against infections. They rapidly respond to foreign invaders, such as bacteria, by engulfing and destroying them through a process called phagocytosis. Neutrophils are crucial for preventing and controlling infections.
2. ***Lymphocytes***: The second most common type, lymphocytes play a vital role in the immune system. They are divided into two main types: B cells and T cells. B cells produce antibodies that specifically target and neutralize viruses, bacteria, and other harmful invaders. T cells, on the other hand, help identify and destroy infected cells and coordinate the overall immune response.
3. ***Monocytes***: The third most common type, monocytes are larger white blood cells that circulate in the bloodstream. When they migrate into tissues, they differentiate into macrophages and dendritic cells.

These cells are essential for engulfing and breaking down pathogens, as well as presenting antigens to T cells, which helps initiate a targeted immune response.

4. ***Eosinophils***: The fourth most common type, eosinophils are particularly effective against parasitic infections, such as those caused by worms. They release toxic granules that can kill parasites and also play a role in modulating the immune response. Eosinophils are also involved in allergic reactions and asthma, where they contribute to inflammation and tissue damage.

5. ***Basophils***: The least common type, basophils are involved in inflammatory reactions and allergic responses. They release histamine and other chemicals that promote inflammation, leading to symptoms such as swelling, redness, and itching. Basophils also play a role in responding to parasitic infections and are important for the regulation of the immune system.

White blood cells are produced in the bone marrow and circulate in the blood and lymphatic system, constantly monitoring for and combating foreign invaders. In CSS, the excessive number of eosinophils leads to inflammation in various parts of the body.

Inflammation is a crucial part of the body's immune response, occurring when the body attempts to heal itself from injury or infection. The main signs and symptoms of inflammation include redness, swelling, heat, and pain. Inflammation can be acute (short-term) or chronic (long-term). Acute inflammation typically lasts for a few days, while chronic inflammation can persist for weeks, months, or even years.

While inflammation is necessary for healing, excessive inflammation can be harmful. Chronic inflammation is linked to several serious health conditions, including heart disease, cancer, and Alzheimer's disease. In CSS, the widespread inflammation of blood vessels can result in significant organ damage.

Symptoms of Churg-Strauss Syndrome (CSS)

The symptoms of Churg-Strauss Syndrome (CSS) can range from mild to severe and may appear suddenly or develop gradually over time. Because CSS affects multiple organs, the symptoms can vary significantly from person to person. The most common symptoms include sinusitis, asthma, and skin problems.

Nearly everyone with CSS (about 95%) experiences sinusitis, which can cause a stuffy or runny nose, facial pain, and tooth pain. Sinusitis is the inflammation of the sinuses, often due to infection, allergies, or other irritants. Common symptoms of sinusitis are headaches, pressure in the sinuses, facial pain, and nasal congestion. While most cases are mild and treatable at home, severe cases may require medical intervention.

Asthma

A history of asthma is also typical among people with Churg-Strauss Syndrome (CSS). Asthma is a chronic lung condition characterized by wheezing, shortness of breath, and chest tightness. It occurs due to inflammation and narrowing of the airways, making breathing difficult. During an asthma attack, the muscles around the airways tighten, and the lining of the airways swells and produces mucus, further obstructing airflow.

Various triggers, such as allergies, cold air, exercise, and stress, can initiate asthma attacks. Pollutants, smoke, and strong odors are also common triggers. Monitoring and avoiding these triggers, along with taking prescribed medications, can help manage asthma symptoms.

Asthma is prevalent, affecting over 25 million people in the United States alone, and is one of the most common chronic conditions in childhood, although it can affect individuals of all ages. The condition can range from mild to severe, with some individuals experiencing only occasional symptoms and others having persistent, daily symptoms that require comprehensive management. Regular check-ups with healthcare providers and personalized action plans are crucial for effective asthma control.

Skin Problems

Skin issues are prevalent in CSS patients, with the most common being rashes, hives, and itching. The rash associated with CSS is typically widespread, and symmetrical, and may fluctuate in severity, often worsening in the morning and improving with activity during the day. This rash can sometimes be accompanied by dryness and cracking of the skin, which can exacerbate discomfort.

Hives are raised, red, itchy welts that can appear anywhere on the body, frequently triggered by allergies. These welts can vary in size and may join together to form larger areas of swelling. They often appear suddenly and can be quite distressing due to their unpredictable nature.

Itching can be severe and may be either widespread or localized to specific areas. This persistent itching can lead to complications such as skin infections from excessive scratching. Managing these symptoms often requires a combination of medications, such as antihistamines, and lifestyle adjustments to avoid known triggers. Regular consultation with a healthcare provider is crucial for effective management of these skin problems.

Other Symptoms

Additional symptoms of CSS include:

- *Fatigue*: Patients with CSS may experience persistent fatigue, which can greatly impact their quality of life.

This fatigue is often related to the body's ongoing inflammatory response and can be managed through proper medication and rest.
- *Weight loss*: Unintentional weight loss is a common symptom in CSS patients, likely due to decreased appetite and increased metabolic demands from chronic inflammation.
- *Fever*: Some individuals with CSS may experience low-grade fevers that come and go. These fevers are typically not dangerous but should still be monitored by a healthcare provider.
- *Joint pain*: Inflammation caused by CSS can also affect the joints, leading to pain, stiffness, and swelling. This can make everyday tasks challenging and affect overall mobility.
- *Nerve problems*: In rare cases, CSS can cause nerve damage, leading to symptoms such as numbness, tingling, or weakness in the arms or legs. This is more commonly seen in severe cases of CSS.

These symptoms arise due to the widespread inflammation and organ involvement characteristic of CSS, emphasizing the need for personalized treatment and management plans for affected individuals.

Causes of Churg-Strauss Syndrome

Churg-Strauss Syndrome, also known as Eosinophilic Granulomatosis with Polyangiitis (EGPA), is a rare autoimmune disorder characterized by inflammation of small to medium-sized blood vessels. The exact cause of Churg-Strauss Syndrome is not known.

However, several factors are believed to contribute to its development:

Genetic Factors

Genetic predispositions may play a significant role in the development of EGPA (Eosinophilic Granulomatosis with Polyangiitis), as certain genetic markers have been linked to an increased risk. Studies have identified specific gene variations that may contribute to the likelihood of developing this condition, indicating a hereditary component.

Immune System Abnormalities

Abnormal immune responses, including the overproduction of eosinophils (a type of white blood cell), can lead to inflammation and damage of blood vessels. This excessive immune activity can cause chronic inflammation, leading to the symptoms associated with EGPA such as asthma, sinusitis, and neuropathy. The exact mechanisms that trigger these immune abnormalities are still under investigation.

Environmental Triggers

Environmental factors such as infections, allergens, or exposure to certain chemicals may trigger the onset of the disease in genetically predisposed individuals. For example, seasonal allergens or fungal spores could exacerbate immune responses in sensitive individuals, potentially initiating the disease process. Additionally, viral or bacterial infections may serve as catalysts that activate the underlying genetic predispositions.

Medications

In some cases, the use of asthma or allergy medications, particularly leukotriene inhibitors and inhaled steroids, has been associated with the development of EGPA, though this is rare. Patients using these medications should be monitored for any unusual symptoms that might indicate the onset of EGPA. The exact relationship between these medications and EGPA is complex and warrants further research.

Pre-existing Conditions

A history of asthma or allergic rhinitis is common among individuals who develop Churg-Strauss Syndrome (another name for EGPA), suggesting a link between these conditions and the syndrome. Asthma, particularly when severe or poorly controlled, is often a precursor to EGPA, indicating that chronic respiratory issues may contribute to the syndrome's development. Managing these pre-existing conditions effectively could potentially reduce the risk of progression to EGPA.

Understanding the exact interplay of these factors remains a subject of ongoing research. However, it is clear that Churg-Strauss Syndrome is a complex and multifactorial disease, making personalized treatment plans crucial for effective management.

Diagnosis

To diagnose Churg-Strauss Syndrome (Eosinophilic Granulomatosis with Polyangiitis), a healthcare provider typically conducts a comprehensive physical examination and reviews the patient's medical history. Additionally, various tests are ordered to confirm the diagnosis and rule out other similar conditions. Here is an overview of the diagnostic approach:

1. **Physical Examination and Medical History**
    - Thorough Physical Exam: Conducting a comprehensive evaluation to identify signs such as skin rashes, breathing difficulties, and nerve problems. This may involve checking vital signs, listening to the heart and lungs, and inspecting the skin for any abnormalities.
    - Medical History Review: Assessing a patient's symptoms, including asthma, allergies, or nasal polyps, and documenting any history of

autoimmune disorders. This review helps to understand the patient's overall health background and any potential underlying conditions that could influence their current state.

2. **Laboratory Tests**
   - ***Complete Blood Count (CBC)***: This test is used to check for elevated eosinophil levels (eosinophilia), which is a hallmark of the syndrome. Eosinophils are a type of white blood cell that becomes elevated in response to certain conditions, including allergies and infections.
   - ***Erythrocyte Sedimentation Rate (ESR) and C-reactive protein (CRP)***: These markers are measured to indicate inflammation in the body. ESR measures how quickly red blood cells settle at the bottom of a test tube, while CRP is a protein produced by the liver in response to inflammation.
   - ***Antineutrophil Cytoplasmic Antibodies (ANCA)***: Specifically looking for p-ANCA; while not always present, it supports the diagnosis if found. ANCA are antibodies that target proteins in the cytoplasm of neutrophils, a type of white blood cell. The presence of p-ANCA can help in diagnosing certain autoimmune disorders.

3. **Imaging Studies**
    - ***Chest X-ray or CT Scan***: Utilized to detect a range of lung abnormalities, such as transient or permanent infiltrates, which may indicate infections like pneumonia, inflammation, or other pathological conditions affecting the lung tissues. These imaging techniques help in visualizing the structure of the lungs, identifying tumors, fibrosis, and other pulmonary issues, and providing a comprehensive overview crucial for diagnosis and treatment planning.
    - ***Sinus Imaging***: Employed to assess for conditions like chronic sinusitis or sinus inflammation, which can cause persistent nasal congestion, facial pain, headaches, and other sinus-related symptoms. Techniques such as X-rays, CT scans, or MRI can provide detailed images of the sinuses, helping doctors to identify blockages, infections, or anatomical abnormalities that may require medical or surgical intervention.
4. **Biopsy**
    - ***Tissue Biopsy***: This involves taking samples from affected areas, such as the skin, lungs, or nerves, which are then meticulously examined under a microscope. The primary focus is to

identify eosinophilic granulomas and vasculitis, key indicators of this syndrome. These findings help in confirming the diagnosis and guiding the subsequent treatment plan.

Diagnostic Criteria

The American College of Rheumatology (ACR) has set criteria for diagnosing Churg-Strauss Syndrome, where meeting at least four of the six following criteria strongly suggests the diagnosis:

1. **Asthma**

    Chronic, often severe asthma can lead to frequent episodes of wheezing, shortness of breath, chest tightness, and persistent coughing. These symptoms are particularly pronounced at night or in the early morning, disrupting sleep and daily activities. Management typically involves long-term medication use, such as inhaled corticosteroids, and monitoring to prevent exacerbations.

2. **Eosinophilia**

    Greater than 10% eosinophils in peripheral blood, indicate an elevated white blood cell count. This condition can be associated with various allergic reactions, infections, or diseases like asthma and eosinophilic esophagitis. Eosinophilia often requires further investigation to identify the underlying cause and appropriate treatment, which might include corticosteroids or other immunosuppressive therapies.

3. **Mononeuropathy or Polyneuropathy**

   Nerve damage symptoms such as numbness, tingling, or weakness, can affect a single nerve (mononeuropathy) or multiple nerves (polyneuropathy). These conditions can lead to significant functional impairments, affecting mobility and the ability to perform daily tasks.

   Causes may include diabetes, autoimmune diseases, or infections, and treatment typically involves addressing the underlying cause, pain management, and physical therapy.

4. **Pulmonary Infiltrates**

   Nonfixed lung infiltrates are detected on imaging, which may appear as cloudy areas on a chest X-ray or CT scan. These infiltrates are indicative of various conditions, including infections like pneumonia, inflammation, or interstitial lung diseases such as sarcoidosis.

   Diagnosis and management often involve further tests, such as sputum cultures, blood tests, or biopsies, and may require antibiotics, steroids, or other treatments depending on the underlying condition.

5. **Paranasal Sinus Abnormality**

   Chronic sinus infections or inflammation that cause symptoms such as nasal congestion, facial pain, pressure, and a reduced sense of smell. These abnormalities often require long-term management strategies, including nasal corticosteroids, saline irrigations, antibiotics for bacterial infections, or surgery in severe cases to improve sinus drainage and function.

6. **Extravascular Eosinophils**

   Eosinophils are found in tissue outside blood vessels, usually identified via biopsy. This finding can signal conditions like eosinophilic granulomatosis with polyangiitis (EGPA) or other eosinophil-associated diseases.

   These conditions can cause a range of symptoms depending on the affected organs, such as skin rashes, gastrointestinal issues, or heart problems. Treatment generally involves immunosuppressive drugs, such as corticosteroids or biologics, to reduce eosinophil levels and manage symptoms.

Combining these diagnostic tools and criteria helps healthcare providers accurately diagnose Churg-Strauss Syndrome and distinguish it from other conditions with similar symptoms.

Treatment of Churg-Strauss Syndrome

The treatment of Churg-Strauss Syndrome (CSS) usually involves a combination of corticosteroids and immunosuppressive drugs.

Corticosteroids

Corticosteroids are anti-inflammatory medications that help reduce inflammation in the blood vessels. These hormones, produced naturally by the body, are involved in various processes such as stress response, immunity, and inflammation.

They can also be synthesized in a laboratory to treat conditions like allergies, asthma, and arthritis. While generally safe when used as directed, corticosteroids can cause serious side effects if not used correctly. It is essential to discuss the risks and benefits with your doctor before starting any treatment.

Immunosuppressive Drugs

Immunosuppressive drugs suppress the immune system to prevent it from attacking the blood vessels. These medications are typically used in people who have had an organ transplant and need to take them for life. Several types of immunosuppressive drugs work differently, including:

- Tacrolimus (Astagraf XL, Prograf)
- Sirolimus (Rapamune)
- Mycophenolate mofetil (CellCept)
- Azathioprine (Imuran)
- Cyclosporine (Neoral, Sandimmune)

Each transplant recipient is prescribed a specific regimen based on individual needs, with the exact combination and dosage potentially varying over time. Common side effects of immunosuppressive drugs include nausea, vomiting, diarrhea, headache, dizziness, trouble sleeping, rash, weight changes, acne, and high blood pressure.

In some cases, surgery might be necessary to repair damaged organs. For example, surgery may be required to repair a heart valve damaged by CSS.

Lifestyle Changes to Manage Churg-Strauss Syndrome

Managing Churg-Strauss Syndrome, also known as Eosinophilic Granulomatosis with Polyangiitis (EGPA), typically involves both medical treatment and lifestyle changes. While it's crucial to work closely with healthcare providers for personalized advice, here are some general lifestyle changes that may help manage the condition:

1. **Medication Adherence**
    - ***Strictly follow medication plans***: Ensure you take prescribed medications, such as corticosteroids and immunosuppressants, exactly as directed by your healthcare provider. This helps manage your symptoms effectively and prevents potential complications.
    - ***Avoid self-medicating***: Always consult your doctor before making any changes to your medication regimen. Self-medicating can lead to adverse reactions or interactions with other drugs you may be taking. Your healthcare provider can guide you on the best course of action.
2. **Regular Medical Check-Ups**
    - ***Frequent monitoring***: Regular check-ups with your healthcare provider are essential to monitor disease activity and adjust treatments as needed. These visits allow your doctor to observe any changes in your condition, ensuring that your treatment plan remains effective and addressing any new symptoms promptly.
    - ***Blood tests and imaging***: Periodic blood tests and imaging studies can help track inflammation levels and organ function. Blood tests can reveal important details about your overall health, such as white blood cell counts

and markers of inflammation. Imaging studies like MRIs or X-rays provide a clear picture of how your organs and tissues are functioning and if there are any areas of concern that need further attention.

3. **Healthy Diet**
   - ***Balanced nutrition***: Emphasize a diet rich in a variety of colorful fruits, vegetables, lean proteins like chicken and fish, and whole grains such as brown rice and quinoa. This helps provide essential vitamins and minerals.
   - ***Limit salt intake***: Reducing salt can help manage blood pressure and reduce the risk of heart disease, especially if corticosteroids are part of your treatment. Opt for herbs and spices to flavor your food instead.
   - ***Stay hydrated***: Drink plenty of water throughout the day to maintain optimal hydration levels. Aim for at least 8 cups of water daily, and consider increasing your intake if you are active or live in a hot climate.

4. **Physical Activity**
   - ***Regular exercise***: Engage in moderate physical activities tailored to your abilities and energy levels, such as walking, swimming, or light aerobics. Consistency is key to maintaining overall health and well-being.

- *Avoid overexertion*: Balance exercise with adequate rest to prevent fatigue and flare-ups. Listen to your body and take breaks when needed to ensure you don't push yourself too hard.

5. **Stress Management**
   - *Mindfulness and relaxation*: Practices like meditation, yoga, and deep-breathing exercises can help reduce stress by calming the mind and promoting a sense of well-being. These activities can be done daily and are particularly effective when integrated into a regular routine.
   - *Adequate sleep*: Aim for 7-9 hours of quality sleep each night to aid in physical recovery and immune function, as well as to improve cognitive performance and emotional stability. Establishing a consistent sleep schedule and creating a restful sleep environment are key factors in achieving good sleep.

6. **Avoiding Triggers**
   - *Environmental factors*: Identify and avoid potential allergens or irritants that could trigger symptoms.
   - *Infection prevention*: Practice good hygiene and stay up-to-date with vaccinations to minimize infection risks.

7. **Support Systems**
   - ***Seek support***: Engage with support groups or counseling to share experiences and receive emotional support.
   - ***Educate family and friends***: Helping those around you understand the condition can foster a supportive environment.

8. **Smoking and Alcohol**
   - ***Quit smoking***: Smoking can exacerbate respiratory symptoms and interfere with overall health.
   - ***Limit alcohol***: Alcohol can interact with medications and affect liver function.

9. **Monitor Symptoms**
   - ***Keep a symptom diary***: Track symptoms and triggers to help identify patterns and inform your healthcare provider.
   - ***Prompt reporting***: Report new or worsening symptoms to your doctor immediately.

Implementing these lifestyle changes can complement medical treatments and help manage Churg-Strauss Syndrome more effectively. Always work closely with your healthcare team to develop a comprehensive management plan tailored to your specific needs.

The 3 Phases of CSS

The onset of CSS is often gradual, with symptoms developing over time. The course of the disease can be divided into three phases:

Phase 1: Prodromal Phase

The prodromal phase, or the initial stage of Churg-Strauss Syndrome (CSS), is when the first symptoms appear. The term "prodromal" signifies a precursor or warning, indicating the onset of the disease. During this phase, individuals may experience a variety of symptoms that can often be mistaken for other conditions.

Symptoms During the Prodromal Phase

1. **Sinus Infections**

   Chronic or recurrent sinus infections are common during this phase. Individuals might suffer from nasal congestion, postnasal drip, and frequent sinus headaches.

2. **Asthma Attacks**

   Asthma is a hallmark symptom of CSS and often develops during the prodromal phase. Patients may experience shortness of breath, wheezing, and frequent asthma attacks. For some, asthma can become severe and persistent, requiring ongoing treatment and management.

3. **Skin Rashes**

   Skin manifestations, such as rashes, are also prevalent. These rashes can appear as red, raised patches or bumps on the skin, often causing discomfort and itching.

4. **Fatigue:**

   Persistent fatigue is a common complaint. This extreme tiredness can affect daily activities and reduce overall quality of life.

5. **Muscle Aches (Myalgia):**

   Muscle aches or myalgia can occur, causing pain and discomfort in various muscle groups. This symptom may be generalized or localized to specific areas.

6. **Joint Pain (Arthralgia):**

   Joint pain, or arthralgia, is another frequent symptom during the prodromal phase. This pain can affect different joints and may be accompanied by swelling and stiffness.

7. **Asthma Development:**

   During the prodromal phase, asthma may develop or worsen if already present. Asthma symptoms include:

   - ***Shortness of Breath***: Difficulty breathing, especially during physical activity or at night.
   - ***Wheezing***: A high-pitched whistling sound when breathing.
   - ***Frequent Asthma Attacks***: Episodes of acute asthma symptoms requiring immediate medical attention.

Recognizing the symptoms during the prodromal phase is crucial for early diagnosis and treatment of CSS. Early intervention can help manage symptoms more effectively and potentially prevent further progression of the disease. If you or someone you know experiences these symptoms persistently, it is important to seek medical advice for appropriate diagnosis and treatment.

Phase 2: Eosinophilic Phase

The second phase of Churg-Strauss Syndrome (CSS) is known as the eosinophilic phase. During this phase, there is a significant increase in eosinophils, a type of white blood cell that plays an essential role in the body's immune response, especially in combating parasitic infections and contributing to allergic reactions.

Characteristics of the Eosinophilic Phase

Eosinophilia: Eosinophils are typically present in small quantities in the blood; however, during the eosinophilic phase, their numbers rise dramatically. This condition, known as eosinophilia, is a hallmark of this phase and can be detected through blood tests.

Symptoms Associated with Eosinophilia:

1. *Fever*: Many patients experience unexplained fevers during this phase. These fevers can be persistent and may not respond well to typical fever-reducing medications.
2. *Weight Loss*: Unintentional weight loss is common, often due to the underlying inflammation and the body's heightened metabolic state while fighting off the perceived threats mediated by eosinophils.
3. *Skin Rash*: Similar to the prodromal phase, skin rashes can persist or worsen. The rashes may present as red, raised patches or plaques on the skin, and might be itchy or painful. Eosinophils can infiltrate the skin, leading to these dermatological manifestations.
4. *Muscle Aches and Pains (Myalgia)*: Muscle aches and pains are prominent during this phase. The increased activity of eosinophils can lead to inflammation in the

muscle tissues, resulting in widespread discomfort and pain.

Additional Symptoms and Complications

In addition to the primary symptoms, the eosinophilic phase can lead to more severe complications due to the infiltration of various organs by eosinophils. These complications include:

1. *Gastrointestinal Symptoms*: Abdominal pain, nausea, vomiting, and diarrhea can occur if eosinophils infiltrate the digestive tract. This can sometimes be mistaken for other gastrointestinal disorders.
2. *Pulmonary Symptoms*: The lungs can be significantly affected, leading to symptoms such as coughing, shortness of breath, and even pulmonary infiltrates visible on chest X-rays.
3. *Cardiac Involvement*: Although rarer, eosinophils can infiltrate the heart, causing conditions like myocarditis (inflammation of the heart muscle), which can lead to chest pain, heart palpitations, and in severe cases, heart failure.
4. *Neurological Symptoms*: Neurological involvement can manifest as peripheral neuropathy, characterized by numbness, tingling, and weakness in the limbs due to nerve damage caused by eosinophilic infiltration.

The eosinophilic phase is critical in the progression of CSS and requires careful monitoring and treatment. Elevated eosinophil levels can cause significant tissue damage and organ dysfunction if not managed promptly.

Treatment typically involves corticosteroids and immunosuppressive drugs to reduce inflammation and control eosinophil levels. Regular follow-up with healthcare providers is essential to monitor the disease's progress and adjust treatment as necessary.

Early recognition and intervention during the eosinophilic phase can significantly improve outcomes and help prevent severe complications associated with Churg-Strauss Syndrome.

Phase 3: Vasculitic Phase

The third and final phase of Churg-Strauss Syndrome (CSS) is known as the vasculitic phase. During this stage, the patient's blood vessels become inflamed, a condition referred to as vasculitis. This phase is particularly critical due to the high risk of serious complications.

Characteristics of the Vasculitic Phase

Vasculitis: Vasculitis refers to inflammation of the blood vessels, which can affect arteries, veins, and capillaries throughout the body. This inflammation can cause the walls of the blood vessels to thicken, reducing the width of the passageway through which blood flows. In severe cases, it can lead to vessel blockage, causing tissue and organ damage.

Serious Complications
1. *Stroke*: Inflammation of the blood vessels in the brain can lead to reduced blood flow or hemorrhage, resulting in a stroke. Symptoms may include sudden weakness, confusion, difficulty speaking, vision problems, and severe headaches.
2. *Heart Attack*: If the coronary arteries are affected, the reduced blood flow can lead to a heart attack. Symptoms often include chest pain, shortness of breath, nausea, and sweating.
3. *Organ Damage*: Various organs can be affected by impaired blood flow, leading to significant damage. The kidneys, lungs, liver, and gastrointestinal tract are among the organs that can suffer due to decreased oxygen and nutrient supply.
4. *Nerve Damage (Peripheral Neuropathy)*: One of the complications of CSS during this phase is nerve damage, also known as peripheral neuropathy. This can occur due to inflammation and damage to the small blood vessels that supply nerves.

Symptoms of Nerve Damage
- *Numbness*: A loss of sensation in the extremities.

- *Tingling*: A prickling or "pins and needles" sensation in the hands and feet.
- *Weakness*: Loss of strength in the muscles controlled by the affected nerves.
- *Paralysis*: In severe cases, complete loss of muscle function in certain areas.

Aggressive Treatment

Due to the high risk of serious complications, treatment during the vasculitic phase is typically very aggressive. The primary goals are to reduce inflammation and prevent further damage to the blood vessels and organs.

Treatment Strategies

- *Corticosteroids*: High doses of corticosteroids are often used to quickly reduce inflammation.
- *Immunosuppressive Drugs*: Medications such as cyclophosphamide, azathioprine, or methotrexate may be used to suppress the immune system and decrease inflammation.
- *Biologic Agents*: Newer treatments may include biologic agents like rituximab, which target specific components of the immune system.
- *Monitoring and Supportive Care*: Patients require close monitoring for signs of complications. Supportive care may include treatments to manage symptoms and maintain organ function.

- ***Physical Therapy***: For those experiencing nerve damage, physical therapy may help improve mobility and strength.

Early recognition and aggressive treatment during the vasculitic phase are crucial to managing Churg-Strauss Syndrome effectively. Continuous medical follow-up is necessary to adjust treatments, monitor for complications, and address any new symptoms promptly. Successful management of this phase can significantly improve outcomes and quality of life for individuals with CSS.

Management Through Diet

There is no specific diet for people with Churg-Strauss Syndrome (CSS), but eating a healthy diet is important for everyone. This chapter will outline general dietary guidelines to help manage the condition and support overall health.

A Balanced, Nutritious Diet

A healthy diet includes a variety of fruits, vegetables, whole grains, and lean proteins. These components are essential for maintaining good health and supporting your body's immune system:

- *Fruits and Vegetables*: Aim for a colorful assortment of fruits and vegetables daily. They are rich in vitamins, minerals, and antioxidants that can help reduce inflammation.
- *Whole Grains*: Choose whole grains like brown rice, oats, and quinoa over refined grains. Whole grains provide fiber, which aids digestion and helps maintain stable blood sugar levels.

- ***Lean Proteins***: Incorporate sources of lean protein such as fish, poultry, beans, and legumes. Protein is crucial for muscle repair and overall body function.

Limiting Unhealthy Fats

It is also important to limit your intake of saturated fats, trans fats, and cholesterol. These substances can contribute to heart disease and other chronic conditions:

- ***Saturated Fats***: Found in fatty cuts of meat, butter, and full-fat dairy products. Choose lower-fat dairy options and leaner cuts of meat to reduce intake.
- ***Trans Fats***: Often found in processed and fried foods. Read labels carefully and avoid products that contain "partially hydrogenated oils."
- ***Cholesterol***: Present in animal products like meat and dairy. Opt for plant-based proteins and lower-cholesterol food options when possible.

Managing Blood Sugar Levels

In addition, because steroids can increase blood sugar levels, it is important to control your intake of sugar and refined carbohydrates. These foods can cause spikes in blood sugar levels, which can be dangerous for people with diabetes:

- ***Refined Carbohydrates***: Foods such as white bread, pastries, and sugary cereals can cause quick spikes in blood sugar. Choose whole-grain alternatives instead.

- ***Sugary Foods and Beverages***: Limit intake of sweets, desserts, and sugary drinks. Opt for natural sweeteners or fruits to satisfy sweet cravings.
- ***Balanced Meals***: Combine carbohydrates with proteins and healthy fats to slow digestion and prevent rapid increases in blood sugar levels.

By following these dietary guidelines, you can help manage the symptoms of Churg-Strauss Syndrome and support your overall health. Always consult with a healthcare provider or a registered dietitian to tailor dietary recommendations specifically to your needs.

5-Step-by-Step Guide to Starting a Diet for Churg-Strauss Syndrome

Although there is no specific diet for Churg-Strauss Syndrome, following a healthy and balanced eating plan can help manage symptoms and support overall health. Here is a 5-step guide to getting started on a diet for Churg-Strauss Syndrome:

Step 1: Consult with Your Healthcare Provider

Begin your journey towards a healthier diet by scheduling a detailed consultation with your healthcare provider. This initial step is essential because Churg-Strauss Syndrome (CSS) is a complex and rare autoimmune condition that can affect multiple systems in your body, including your blood vessels, skin, lungs, heart, and gastrointestinal tract. Given the complexity of CSS, it's crucial to have a healthcare professional guide you through any dietary modifications.

During the consultation, provide a comprehensive overview of your medical history, current symptoms, and any treatments or medications you are currently taking. Be open and detailed about your previous dietary habits and any changes you've already attempted, as this context can help your provider give more precise advice.

Ask specific questions about how diet might influence your condition. For instance, inquire if there are particular foods known to exacerbate CSS symptoms, or if there are beneficial nutrients that you should focus on to help reduce inflammation and support overall health. Your healthcare provider may recommend specific blood tests or other diagnostic measures to identify potential nutritional deficiencies or other issues that could be addressed through diet.

Your healthcare provider may suggest working with a registered dietitian or nutritionist specialized in autoimmune or inflammatory conditions. These experts can create a personalized nutrition plan tailored to your needs, explaining the roles of macronutrients (proteins, fats, and carbs) and micronutrients (vitamins and minerals) in managing inflammation and supporting immune function.

It's crucial to discuss how your diet interacts with any medications you're taking. Some foods can interfere with medication absorption or effectiveness, while others might cause adverse reactions when combined with certain drugs. Your healthcare provider can guide you through these potential issues, ensuring that your dietary changes do not conflict with your treatment.

Remember, this initial consultation is just the start. Schedule regular follow-up appointments to monitor your progress, assess the effectiveness of your dietary changes, and make necessary adjustments. Ongoing collaboration with your healthcare team will be key in managing Churg-Strauss Syndrome effectively through diet and lifestyle modifications.

By taking this proactive approach, you can better manage your symptoms, support your overall health, and potentially improve your quality of life in the face of Churg-Strauss Syndrome.

Step 2: Educate Yourself on Anti-Inflammatory Foods

When managing Churg-Strauss Syndrome, a crucial step is to educate yourself on anti-inflammatory foods. This autoimmune condition involves the inflammation of blood vessels, making it essential to focus on a diet that can help reduce inflammation.

1. **Fruits and Vegetables**

    Incorporate a variety of fruits and vegetables into your meals. These are rich in antioxidants, vitamins, and minerals that combat inflammation. Berries like blueberries, strawberries, and raspberries are especially high in antioxidants. Leafy greens such as spinach, kale, and Swiss chard are also excellent choices due to their high levels of vitamins A, C, and K.

2. Whole Grains

Switch to whole grains instead of refined grains. Whole grains like brown rice, quinoa, and oats have more fiber and nutrients, which can help regulate your immune system and reduce inflammation. Avoiding processed and refined carbohydrates can prevent spikes in blood sugar, which are linked to increased inflammatory markers.

3. Lean Proteins

Lean proteins should be a staple in your diet. Opt for sources like chicken, turkey, tofu, and legumes, which provide essential amino acids without the saturated fats found in red meat. Reducing saturated fat intake is important because it can exacerbate inflammation.

4. Healthy Fats

Healthy fats are vital for combating inflammation. Incorporate foods rich in omega-3 fatty acids, such as salmon, mackerel, sardines, and flaxseeds. These fats have been shown to lower inflammation and improve overall heart health. Additionally, using olive oil as your primary cooking oil can provide monounsaturated fats that support a healthy inflammatory response.

Additional Tips

- *Nuts and Seeds*: Incorporate nuts like almonds and walnuts, and seeds like chia and hemp seeds, which are packed with healthy fats, protein, and fiber.
- *Spices and Herbs*: Use anti-inflammatory spices like turmeric, ginger, and garlic in your cooking. These not only add flavor but also offer potent anti-inflammatory benefits.
- *Hydration*: Stay well-hydrated by drinking plenty of water throughout the day. Proper hydration helps maintain bodily functions and can aid in reducing inflammation.

By focusing on these dietary changes, you can help manage the symptoms of Churg-Strauss Syndrome more effectively. Always consult with a healthcare provider or a nutritionist before making significant changes to your diet, especially when dealing with a complex condition like this.

Step 3: Plan Balanced Meals

Creating a balanced meal plan is essential for managing Churg-Strauss Syndrome and sustaining overall health. A well-rounded diet ensures you get all the necessary nutrients to support your body's functions, reduce inflammation, and maintain steady energy levels throughout the day. Here's how to effectively plan your meals:

1. **Nutrient-Dense Foods**

   Focus on incorporating a variety of nutrient-dense foods into your diet. These are foods that offer high levels of vitamins, minerals, and other essential nutrients without excessive calories. They help in maintaining optimal health and can contribute significantly to reducing inflammation.

2. **Balanced Macronutrients**

   Each meal should be a balanced mix of macronutrients: proteins, carbohydrates, and fats. This balance helps to stabilize blood sugar levels, provide sustained energy, and support muscle repair and growth.

   - *Proteins*: Proteins are crucial for tissue repair and immune function. Include lean sources such as chicken, turkey, fish, eggs, tofu, legumes, and low-fat dairy products.
   - *Carbohydrates*: Carbohydrates provide the primary source of energy. Opt for complex carbohydrates like whole grains, vegetables, and fruits, which release energy slowly and help keep blood sugar levels stable.

- *Fats*: Healthy fats are important for hormone production and reducing inflammation. Incorporate sources like avocados, nuts, seeds, olive oil, and fatty fish (rich in omega-3 fatty acids).

3. **Portion Sizes**

    Pay close attention to portion sizes to avoid overeating and ensure you're getting the right amount of nutrients. Using a balanced plate method can be helpful:

    - Fill half your plate with fruits and vegetables.
    - Allocate one-quarter of the plate to lean proteins.
    - Use the remaining quarter for whole grains or starchy vegetables.

4. **Regular Eating Intervals**

    Eating at regular intervals is crucial to maintaining steady energy levels. Aim for three main meals and two snacks per day. This approach helps prevent energy dips and keeps your metabolism active.

Sample Meal Plan

Here's a sample meal plan to demonstrate how to structure balanced meals throughout the day:

- *Breakfast*: Greek yogurt with mixed berries, a sprinkle of chia seeds, and a drizzle of honey. Add a slice of whole-grain toast with avocado.

- *Mid-Morning Snack*: An apple with a handful of almonds.
- *Lunch*: Grilled chicken breast over a quinoa salad with mixed greens, cherry tomatoes, cucumbers, and a lemon-olive oil vinaigrette.
- *Afternoon Snack*: Hummus with carrot and celery sticks.
- *Dinner*: Baked salmon with a side of roasted sweet potatoes and steamed broccoli tossed in olive oil and garlic.
- *Evening Snack*: A small bowl of mixed fruit or a few squares of dark chocolate.

By planning balanced meals with these guidelines, you can ensure that your body gets a steady supply of energy and nutrients throughout the day. Always consider consulting with a healthcare provider or a nutritionist to tailor your meal plan to your specific needs and health conditions.

Step 4: Monitor and Adjust

Maintaining a proactive approach to managing Churg-Strauss Syndrome involves closely monitoring your diet and its impact on your symptoms. By keeping a food diary, you can gain valuable insights into how different foods affect your condition, allowing you to make informed adjustments for better health outcomes. Here's how to effectively monitor and adjust your diet:

1. **Keeping a Food Diary**

   A food diary is an essential tool for tracking your dietary intake and identifying potential triggers for flare-ups. It should include detailed records of what you eat and drink, along with notes on portion sizes, meal times, and any symptoms experienced.

   <u>What to Record</u>

   - ***Daily Intake***: Document every meal, snack, and beverage consumed throughout the day.
   - ***Portion Sizes***: Note approximate portion sizes to help identify patterns in your intake.
   - ***Meal Times***: Record the time of each meal and snack to track eating intervals.
   - ***Symptoms***: Write down any symptoms experienced, such as fatigue, pain, or gastrointestinal issues, noting their severity and timing.
   - ***Additional Factors***: Include any other relevant factors that might affect your condition, such as stress levels, physical activity, and sleep quality.

2. **How to Use Your Food Diary**
   - ***Identify Patterns***: Regularly review your diary to spot any correlations between specific foods and symptom changes. Look for patterns that suggest certain foods may be beneficial or problematic.

- ***Track Progress***: Monitor improvements or exacerbations in your condition over time. This helps assess the effectiveness of dietary changes and informs future adjustments.
- ***Consult Professionals***: Share your food diary with healthcare providers or nutritionists. Their expertise can help interpret the data and provide personalized dietary recommendations.

3. Making Adjustments

Based on the observations from your food diary, you may need to make adjustments to your diet to better manage Churg-Strauss Syndrome.

Identifying Triggers

- ***Common Triggers***: Certain foods are more likely to trigger inflammation or allergic reactions. Common triggers include processed foods, sugary snacks, and foods high in saturated fats.
- ***Personal Triggers***: Everyone's body reacts differently. Use your diary to pinpoint foods that specifically exacerbate your symptoms.

4. Implementing Changes

- ***Eliminate Triggers***: Gradually remove identified trigger foods from your diet to see if symptoms improve. Avoid abrupt changes, as they can be difficult to sustain.

- **Introduce Alternatives**: Replace trigger foods with healthier alternatives. For example, swap processed snacks with fresh fruits or nuts.
- **Maintain Balance**: Ensure that any dietary changes still result in balanced meals with adequate nutrients. Seek guidance from a nutritionist to avoid nutritional deficiencies.

5. **Continuous Monitoring**
- **Regular Updates**: Keep updating your food diary even after making initial adjustments. Continuous monitoring ensures long-term management of your condition.
- **Reassess Periodically**: Every few months, reassess your diet and symptoms to determine if further adjustments are needed. Conditions and dietary responses can change over time.

By diligently tracking your diet and symptoms, and making thoughtful adjustments based on this data, you can better manage Churg-Strauss Syndrome. This ongoing process requires dedication but can lead to significant improvements in your quality of life. Always involve healthcare professionals in your journey to ensure safe and effective dietary management.

Step 5: Stay Hydrated and Limit Processed Foods

Maintaining proper hydration is essential for maintaining overall health, but it is especially important for those with Churg-Strauss Syndrome. Hydration helps flush out toxins and reduce inflammation in the body. Aim to drink at least 8 glasses of water a day and limit your intake of processed foods, which are often high in sodium and can contribute to inflammation.

Processed foods also tend to lack key nutrients and may worsen symptoms over time. Instead, opt for whole, unprocessed foods as much as possible.

In addition to staying hydrated and eating a balanced diet, regular exercise and stress management techniques can also help improve overall health and manage symptoms of Churg-Strauss Syndrome. Consult with your healthcare team for personalized recommendations on incorporating these practices into your routine.

Foods to Avoid

When managing Churg-Strauss Syndrome (CSS), it's important to focus on a balanced diet that supports overall health and avoids foods that can exacerbate symptoms or interfere with medications. Here are some foods to consider avoiding:

1. **High-Sugar Foods**
    - Sugary Beverages: Sodas, energy drinks, sweetened teas, and fruit juices.
    - Sweets and Desserts: Candy, pastries, cookies, cakes, and ice cream.
    - Refined Sugars: Items with added sugars, such as certain cereals and flavored yogurts.
2. **Refined Carbohydrates**
    - White Bread: Opt for whole-grain alternatives instead.
    - Pasta and Rice: Choose whole-grain versions over refined options.
    - Processed Snacks: Crackers, chips, and other processed snack foods that are high in refined carbohydrates.
3. **Saturated and Trans Fats**
    - Fried Foods: French fries, fried chicken, and other deep-fried items.
    - Fast Food: Many fast food items are high in unhealthy fats.
    - Full-Fat Dairy Products: Whole milk, full-fat cheese, and butter.
    - Processed Meats: Sausages, bacon, and other high-fat, processed meats.
    - Margarine and Shortening: Often contain trans fats.

4. **High-Cholesterol Foods**
    - Organ Meats: Liver and other organ meats that are high in cholesterol.
    - Shellfish: Certain shellfish have high cholesterol content.
    - Egg Yolks: Limit intake if you have cholesterol concerns.
5. **Foods with High Sodium Content**
    - Processed Foods: Canned soups, deli meats, and packaged meals often contain high levels of sodium.
    - Salty Snacks: Pretzels, chips, and salted nuts.
    - Sauces and Condiments: Soy sauce, ketchup, and salad dressings with high sodium content.
6. **Alcohol and Caffeine**
    - Alcoholic Beverages: Can interfere with medications and overall health.
    - High-Caffeine Drinks: Excessive coffee, energy drinks, and other highly caffeinated beverages.
7. **Allergenic or Intolerant Foods**
    - Known Allergens: Foods that you know you are allergic to or have an intolerance for, as they can trigger symptoms.

By avoiding these foods, you can help manage your symptoms more effectively and support your overall health. Always consult with your healthcare provider or a registered dietitian for personalized dietary advice tailored to your specific needs and condition.

Foods to Eat

Managing Churg-Strauss Syndrome (CSS) through diet involves focusing on nutrient-dense foods that support overall health and help manage symptoms. Here are some foods that are generally recommended:

1. **Fruits and Vegetables**
   - *Colorful Variety*: Include a wide range of fruits and vegetables to ensure you get a variety of vitamins, minerals, and antioxidants. Examples include berries, oranges, leafy greens, carrots, and bell peppers.
   - *Anti-Inflammatory Choices*: Foods like berries, cherries, spinach, kale, and broccoli can help reduce inflammation.
2. **Whole Grains**

   Opt for whole-grain bread, brown rice, quinoa, oatmeal, and barley instead of refined grains. These provide fiber, which aids in digestion and helps maintain stable blood sugar levels.

3. **Lean Proteins**
   - *Fish*: Fatty fish like salmon, mackerel, and sardines are rich in omega-3 fatty acids, which have anti-inflammatory properties.
   - *Poultry*: Skinless chicken and turkey are good sources of lean protein.
   - *Legumes*: Beans, lentils, and chickpeas are excellent plant-based protein sources.
   - *Tofu and Tempeh*: These soy products are good alternatives to meat.

4. **Healthy Fats**
   - *Nuts and Seeds*: Almonds, walnuts, chia seeds, and flaxseeds provide healthy fats and fiber.
   - *Avocado*: A source of monounsaturated fats that are good for heart health.
   - *Olive Oil*: Use extra virgin olive oil for cooking and dressings as it is rich in healthy fats.

5. **Dairy Alternatives**

   Low-Fat or Non-Dairy Options: Choose low-fat dairy or non-dairy alternatives like almond milk, soy milk, and yogurt made from coconut or almond milk.

6. **Hydration**
   - *Water*: Drink plenty of water throughout the day to stay hydrated.
   - *Herbal Teas*: Non-caffeinated herbal teas can be soothing and hydrating.

7. **Fiber-Rich Foods**
    - *Vegetables*: Broccoli, Brussels sprouts, and artichokes are high in fiber.
    - *Whole Fruits*: Apples, pears, and berries provide fiber with minimal impact on blood sugar levels.
    - *Whole Grains and Legumes*: As mentioned earlier, these also contribute to your daily fiber intake.
8. **Spices and Herbs**
    - *Anti-Inflammatory Spices*: Incorporate turmeric, ginger, garlic, and cinnamon into your meals for their anti-inflammatory benefits.
    - *Fresh Herbs*: Basil, parsley, cilantro, and thyme can add flavor without adding sodium.

By incorporating these foods into your diet, you can support your overall health and help manage the symptoms of Churg-Strauss Syndrome. Always consult with your healthcare provider or a registered dietitian to ensure your diet meets your specific needs and health goals.

7-Day Meal Plan

Creating a meal plan is a great way for you to start with this diet program that is good for your condition. Creating meal plans may seem challenging at first, but it'll help you with a lot of things in the long run. You can prepare your ingredients beforehand.

You can review each ingredient and find out how each can benefit you. Switching to a healthier, more nutritious diet should be a fun change because you need to stay motivated to stick to this diet to better your health.

The sample 7-day meal plan below can be followed or modified according to your preference or routine.

Day 1

Breakfast: Chia Seed and Strawberry Pudding

Lunch: Salmon with Honey and Mustard

Dinner: Broccoli Soup

Day 2

Breakfast: Tofu Scramble

Lunch: Lentil Stew

Dinner: Cauliflower Pizza

Day 3

Breakfast: Blueberry Flax Smoothie

Lunch: Quinoa-Based Oriental Salad

Dinner: Quinoa Stuffed Peppers

Day 4

Breakfast: Fried Eggs and Vegetables

Lunch: Steamed Cauliflower and Curried Shrimp

Dinner: Low-Cholesterol Waldorf Salad

Day 5

Breakfast: Blueberry Flax Smoothie

Lunch: Udon Salmon Soup

Dinner: Baked Spanish Mackerel Filets

Day 6

Breakfast: Toasted Muesli

Lunch: Baked Spanish Mackerel Filets

Dinner: Quinoa-Based Oriental Salad

Day 7

Breakfast: Chia Seed and Strawberry Pudding

Lunch: Low-Cholesterol Waldorf Salad

Dinner: Steamed Cauliflower and Curried Shrimp

Sample Recipes

Baked Spanish Mackerel Fillets

Ingredients:

- 6 pcs. Spanish mackerel fillets
- 1/4 cup canola oil
- salt
- ground black pepper
- paprika
- 12 slices lemon

Instructions:

1. Arrange the oven rack so that it lies around 6 inches away from the source of heat.
2. Preheat the oven to 500°F.
3. Get a baking dish and lightly grease it.
4. Prepare each mackerel by rubbing both sides with canola oil.
5. Season the filets with salt, pepper, and paprika.
6. Top each filet with a couple of lemon slices.
7. Bake the filets for about 5 to 7 minutes, or just until the fish starts to flake.
8. Serve the fish right away.

Udon Salmon Soup

Ingredients:

- 8 oz. dried udon noodles, may also use ramen or soba, cooked and drained according to package instructions
- 1 clove garlic, smashed and peeled
- 4 oz. cremini mushrooms or button mushrooms, sliced thinly
- 2 scallions, sliced thinly
- 8 oz. salmon fillet, skinned and cut into 1-inch cubes
- 2 tbsp. white miso
- 1 cup boiling water
- 2 cups chicken or vegetable broth, homemade or store-bought, no salt added
- 1/2 tsp. seasoned rice vinegar
- 1 tsp. oyster sauce
- 1/4 tsp. toasted sesame oil

Instructions:

1. Boil a kettle of water.
2. Dissolve the miso in a cup of boiling water.
3. Pour the mixture through a fine-mesh strainer into a heavy saucepan or Dutch oven over medium heat.
4. Add broth, garlic, oyster sauce, and rice vinegar.
5. Once the mixture starts bubbling, reduce the heat to medium-low and cook for 5 minutes.

6. Stir in mushrooms and salmon. Cook for 15 minutes.
7. Remove the saucepan from the heat and stir in scallion, toasted sesame oil, and cooked udon noodles. Discard garlic.
8. Let sit for 3 to 5 minutes before serving.

Steamed Cauliflower and Curried Shrimp

Ingredients:

- 1 whole cauliflower, separated into florets
- 2 tbsp. canola oil
- 2 cloves garlic, minced
- 1 cup sweet peppers, chopped finely
- 1 lb. bay shrimp, pre-cooked
- 1 tsp. curry powder
- 1 tsp. butter
- 3 tbsp. flour
- 1/2 cup fish or vegetable broth
- 2/3 cup milk, low-fat
- 1 tbsp. fresh dill, finely chopped
- 1/4 cup pine nuts, toasted

Instructions:

1. Steam the cauliflower until tender. Set aside.
2. Use a frying pan to sauté the garlic. Add the peppers. Continue cooking until the peppers start to soften.
3. Add the curry powder and the shrimp. Remove pan from heat and set aside.
4. Prepare the roux. Melt the butter. Add the flour and whisk. Heat until the roux becomes light golden brown.

5. Add the milk and broth to the roux gradually. Whisk to incorporate. Stir constantly until the sauce starts to bubble.
6. Add the curried shrimp. Bring the heat down and cook for another 5 minutes.
7. Toss the cauliflower in the shrimp sauce.
8. Transfer to a serving platter. Garnish with dill and pine nuts.

Chia Seed and Strawberry Pudding

Ingredients:

- 1 cup strawberries, thinly sliced
- 3 tbsp. chia seeds
- 1 cup soy beverage, unsweetened and fortified

Instructions:

1. To create pudding, combine the soy beverage and chia seeds. Refrigerate the mixture for half an hour. Stir the mixture every 5 minutes to prevent the chia seeds from sticking together.
2. As an alternative, blend the soy beverage and chia seeds in a food processor and let it chill in the refrigerator.
3. Slice strawberries lengthwise.
4. Pour chilled pudding into 2 glasses. Place the strawberry slices on top.
5. Serve and enjoy your pudding.

Low-Cholesterol Waldorf Salad

Ingredients:

- 1/2 cup raisins
- 2 tbsp. apple-flavored yogurt, fat-free
- 1/2 cup apple juice
- 2 tbsp. mayonnaise, fat-free
- 1 cup celery, finely chopped
- 1/4 cup toasted walnuts, chopped coarsely
- 1 cup apple, chopped

Instructions:

1. Combine apple juice and raisins in a microwavable bowl. Set to high heat in the microwave for thirty seconds.
2. Let it stand for two minutes. Drain.
3. Combine celery, apple, walnuts, and raisins in a bowl.
4. Stir the yogurt and mayonnaise into the mixture.
5. Serve immediately.

Quinoa-Based Oriental Salad

Ingredients:

- 2 cups uncooked quinoa
- 4 cups vegetable broth
- 1 cup edamame
- 1/4 cup chopped green onion
- 1 1/2 tsp. chopped fresh mint
- 1/2 cup chopped carrot
- 1/2 cup chopped red bell pepper
- 1/8 tsp. pepper flakes
- 1/2 tsp. grated orange zest
- 2 tbsp. chopped fresh Thai basil
- Juice from half an orange
- 1 tsp. sesame seeds
- 1 tbsp. sesame oil
- 1 tbsp. olive oil
- 1/8 tsp. black pepper

Instructions:

1. Mix the broth and quinoa in a pan.
2. Set the stove to high and place the pan. Let the mixture heat up for 12 to 14 minutes.
3. After heating, cover the pan and wait for 4 minutes.
4. Place the mixture in a separate container and add the rest of the ingredients.
5. Let it cool down before serving.

Broccoli Soup

Ingredients:

- 1 onion, chopped
- 1 lb. broccoli, chopped
- 1 small tomato, chopped
- 1 tbsp. grapeseed oil
- 1/2 cup unsweetened almond milk
- 16 oz. water
- 1/4 tsp. turmeric
- cayenne pepper, to taste

Instructions:

1. Put oil and onion in a medium pot. Saute over medium heat for about a couple of minutes.
2. Add the seasoning, tomato, and broccoli. Saute for 10 more minutes.
3. Add 6 ounces of water. Cover the pot and let it simmer for a couple more minutes.
4. Transfer the contents into a blender, followed by the remaining water and milk. Blend for a couple of minutes.
5. Pour back the blended ingredients into the pot.
6. Raise up the heat and boil for a couple of minutes.

Blueberry Flax Smoothie

Ingredients:

- 1 cup blueberries, frozen
- 1 tbsp. flaxseed, ground
- a handful of spinach leaves
- 1/4 cup full-fat Greek yogurt
- 1 cup coconut milk or any kind of milk

Instruction:

1. Combine all ingredients in a blender.
2. Blend until smooth and creamy, adding more milk if needed to reach desired consistency.
3. Pour into a glass and enjoy immediately, or store in the refrigerator for later consumption.

Fried Eggs and Vegetables

Ingredients:

- coconut oil
- 1 pack frozen vegetable mix
- 3-4 pcs. eggs
- pepper
- salt
- a few stalks of spinach
- spice mix or preferred spices
- desired fruit

Instructions:

1. Heat a frying pan and pour coconut oil.
2. Add the vegetables.
3. Add eggs, followed by salt, pepper, and spices, according to your taste preference.
4. If using, add spinach.
5. Stir fry until cooked. Don't overcook the vegetables.
6. Serve while warm.

Toasted Muesli

Ingredients:

- 4 cups oats
- 1-1/2 cups raw walnut
- 1/2 cup pepitas
- 1/2 cup raw sunflower seeds
- 1/4 cup honey
- 2 tbsp. olive oil
- 1-1/2 tsp. ground cardamom
- 1/2 tsp. salt
- 1 cup freeze-dried strawberries
- 1 cup freeze-dried blueberries
- non-dairy milk or yogurt

Instructions:

1. Preheat your oven to 300°F (150°C).
2. Combine oats, walnuts, pepitas, sunflower seeds, honey, olive oil, cardamom, and salt in a large bowl. Mix until evenly coated.
3. Spread the mixture on a lined baking sheet.
4. Bake for about 25 minutes or until golden brown and crispy.
5. Let it cool completely before adding freeze-dried strawberries and blueberries.
6. Serve with non-dairy milk or yogurt for a delicious breakfast option that's packed with nutrients!

Lentil Stew

Ingredients:

- 4 cups savoy cabbage, chopped
- 1 tbsp. anchovy paste
- 3-1/2 tbsp. extra virgin olive oil
- 2 tsp. cumin
- 1 shallot, chopped finely
- 1 tsp. turmeric
- 1 leek, chopped finely
- 4 carrots, chopped finely
- 2 celery stalks, chopped finely
- peppered
- unrefined sea salt
- 2 cups organic vegetable broth
- 1 26-oz. can of chopped tomatoes, drained
- 2 15-oz. cans of lentils, rinsed and drained
- 1 tbsp. unfiltered and unpasteurized apple cider vinegar
- 1/2 cup parsley, chopped
- 4 organic pasture-raised eggs
- optional: egg topping

Instructions:

1. Boil water in a large pot.
2. Add cabbage and let cook for about 10 minutes, or until soft. Drain after and set aside.

3. In the same pot, pour in oil and place over medium heat.
4. Add the cumin, anchovy paste, shallots, turmeric, celery, carrots, and leeks.
5. Saute for about 8 to 10 minutes, or until the vegetables are soft.
6. Season with salt and pepper, according to your taste.
7. Add the tomatoes and cabbage, and let cook for another 5 minutes.
8. Pour in the vegetable broth and cook for 10 minutes.
9. Add lentils and cook for another 5 minutes.
10. Remove stew from heat, and add parsley.
11. Serve while hot.

Salmon with Honey and Mustard

Ingredients:

- 3 salmon fillets, patted dry
- pepper
- 2 tbsp. honey
- 1 tbsp. Dijon mustard

Instructions:

1. Create a foil sling for the basket of your air fryer. Both the length and breadth of the foil must be larger than that of the basket. Lay the foil across the basket.
2. Coat the basket and foil with cooking spray.
3. Season them with some pepper.
4. In a small bowl, pour honey and dijon and mix them well. Save a tablespoon of glaze for later. Drizzle the remaining glaze evenly over the fillets.
5. Arrange the fillets in the basket.
6. Cook for 10 minutes at 350°F, until salmon flakes easily.
7. Lift salmon from the air fryer using the sling.
8. Use a spatula to loosen the skin of the fish. Leave the skin behind. Transfer fillets to a plate.
9. Drizzle a reserved gaze over them. Garnish with parsley.
10. Serve them warm.

Cauliflower Pizza

Ingredients:

- cauliflower
- 1/4 cup of tomato pasta sauce
- 1/4 cup of pesto sauce (no sugar)
- 100 grams of thinly sliced mozzarella
- 250 grams of cut tomatoes
- 2-3 medium-sized eggs
- basil leaves

Instructions:

1. Cauliflower-made dough
2. Wash the cauliflower.
3. Roughly chop the washed vegetables.
4. Place the chopped cauliflower into a food processor and pulse until fine-looking.
5. Squeeze any remnants of water from the processed cauliflower
6. Spread the dough over baking trays lined with baking paper.
7. Bake the cauliflower dough for 15 minutes in an oven preheated to 140 C.
8. Let the dough sit and cool down.
9. Place the baked cauliflower in the food processor, with almond meal, oil, parmesan, a pinch of salt and peppers, and eggs.

10. Whiz until smooth.
11. Spread the cauliflower dough in a circular shape on the same pan.
12. Roast at 180°C for 25 minutes.
13. Once done, let it cool for a couple of minutes.
14. Start spreading tomato sauce and half of the pesto sauce.
15. Top it with the mozzarella cheese and then bake it at 250°C for 5-10 minutes until the cheese is melted.
16. While waiting, mix the tomato with the remaining pesto sauce.
17. Put tomatoes and basil on top of the freshly baked pizza.
18. Serve and enjoy while warm.

Quinoa Stuffed Peppers

Ingredients:

- 4 sweet bell peppers, halved vertically, with ribs and seeds removed
- 3/4 cup quinoa, well rinsed
- 15 oz. tomatoes, diced
- 4 cups basil leaves
- 10 oz. baby spinach
- 1 clove garlic, small
- 1/4 cup pistachios, unsalted
- 6 tbsp. grated parmesan cheese
- 3 tbsp. extra-virgin olive oil
- 3 tbsp. boiling water
- 1/4 tsp. kosher salt
- a pinch of black pepper, freshly ground

Instructions:

1. Combine the basil, garlic, parmesan cheese, olive oil, black pepper, and a pinch of salt in a food processor or blender.
2. Blend until the texture of the mixture appears finely chopped.
3. Stir in the boiling water.
4. To make the stuffed peppers:
5. Place the bell pepper halves with the side up on a lightly oiled baking sheet.

6. Roast in the oven using the high setting for about 10 minutes, or until they start to soften and have become slightly charred.
7. Remove the peppers from the oven. Set them aside.
8. In a medium pot, let the quinoa and tomatoes simmer in the vegetable broth for 10 minutes.
9. Stir in the baby spinach in small batches.
10. Scoop the quinoa-spinach mixture. Place them into the roasted peppers.
11. Drizzle the filled bell peppers with the pesto sauce.
12. Garnish with pistachios on top upon serving.

Tofu Scramble

Ingredients:

- 1 block drained tofu, sliced into an inch
- 2-3 tsp. oil
- 1/2 onion, diced
- salt, to taste
- ground black pepper, to taste
- 2/3 cups salsa
- Optional: 2 tsp. nutritional yeast
- Optional: 1/3 tsp. turmeric

Instructions:

1. In a large pan, put the oil and sauté the chopped onion.
2. Add the tofu. Pour out oil if needed, and stir frequently.
3. Add the yeast and turmeric. Stir.
4. When the tofu slices are all coated, add the salsa. Stir frequently.
5. Wait for 1 to 2 minutes for it to be cooked. Season with salt and pepper.
6. Serve while warm.

Conclusion

Thank you for taking the time to read through this comprehensive guide on managing Churg-Strauss Syndrome (CSS). Your interest and dedication to understanding this complex condition are commendable. Navigating life with CSS doesn't come without challenges, but your commitment to learning and applying effective management strategies can make a significant difference in your journey toward better health.

As you've seen throughout this guide, Churg-Strauss Syndrome is a rare and chronic condition characterized by inflammation of blood vessels, which can lead to various symptoms affecting multiple organ systems. While there is currently no cure for Churg-Strauss Syndrome, there are effective ways to manage the symptoms and improve your quality of life. Medication, regular medical check-ups, and lifestyle modifications play critical roles in controlling the disease's progression and minimizing flare-ups.

One crucial aspect of managing CSS involves adopting a healthy diet. A balanced and nutritious diet can support your overall well-being and bolster your body's ability to cope with the condition. Incorporating a variety of nutrient-dense foods can help you maintain energy levels, support your immune system, and reduce inflammation. Fresh fruits, vegetables, lean proteins, whole grains, and healthy fats should form the cornerstone of your daily meals.

It's essential to stay hydrated and avoid foods that may trigger inflammation or exacerbate symptoms. Processed foods, excessive sugar, and saturated fats can potentially worsen inflammation and should be limited. Instead, focus on eating fresh, whole foods that provide your body with essential vitamins and minerals. Omega-3 fatty acids, found in fish, flaxseeds, and walnuts, have anti-inflammatory properties and can be particularly beneficial.

Remember, every individual's experience with CSS is unique, and dietary needs may vary. It's always a good idea to work closely with your healthcare team, including a registered dietitian, to tailor a diet plan that meets your specific requirements and preferences. They can help you identify any food sensitivities or allergies that might be contributing to your symptoms and suggest alternatives to ensure you get the nutrients you need.

Living with Churg-Strauss Syndrome can be overwhelming, but you're not alone. Finding support from healthcare professionals, family, friends, and support groups can provide emotional comfort and practical advice. Sharing your experiences and learning from others who understand what you're going through can be incredibly empowering and reassuring.

Your proactive approach to managing your health is truly inspiring. By educating yourself about Churg-Strauss Syndrome and making informed choices about your lifestyle and diet, you're taking control of your condition rather than letting it control you. Celebrate the small victories and progress you make along the way, and don't be discouraged by setbacks. Every step you take towards better health is a step in the right direction.

In conclusion, while there is no cure for Churg-Strauss Syndrome, effective management strategies and a healthy diet can significantly improve your quality of life. Continue to prioritize your health, seek guidance from your healthcare team, and stay positive. Your journey with CSS is uniquely yours, and with the right tools and support, you can navigate it successfully.

Thank you once again for dedicating your time to reading this guide. Your commitment to understanding and managing Churg-Strauss Syndrome is the first step toward a healthier future. Stay informed, stay encouraged, and remember that you're capable of living a fulfilling life despite the challenges posed by this condition.

FAQs

What are the main goals of managing Churg-Strauss Syndrome?

The primary goals of managing Churg-Strauss Syndrome (CSS) are to control inflammation, prevent organ damage, manage symptoms, and achieve and maintain remission. This involves a combination of medication, lifestyle changes, and regular medical follow-ups.

What medications are typically used in the treatment of Churg-Strauss Syndrome?

Common medications for CSS include corticosteroids to reduce inflammation, immunosuppressive drugs to control the immune system, and biological agents targeting specific components of the immune response. The choice of medication depends on the severity and specific manifestations of the disease.

Can diet play a role in managing Churg-Strauss Syndrome?

Yes, a healthy diet can support overall well-being and help manage symptoms. Eating a balanced diet rich in anti-inflammatory foods, such as fresh fruits, vegetables, whole grains, lean proteins, and healthy fats, can be beneficial. Avoiding processed foods, excessive sugars, and saturated fats may also help reduce inflammation.

How important is it to remain physically active with Churg-Strauss Syndrome?

Regular physical activity is important for maintaining overall health and well-being. Exercise can help improve cardiovascular health, reduce stress, and enhance mood. It's essential to work with your healthcare provider to develop an exercise plan that considers your specific condition and limitations.

What are some strategies for managing daily symptoms of Churg-Strauss Syndrome?

Effective symptom management strategies include taking prescribed medications consistently, following a healthy diet, staying hydrated, getting regular exercise, managing stress through techniques like mindfulness or yoga, and avoiding known triggers such as allergens or certain medications. Regular medical check-ups are also crucial.

How often should someone with Churg-Strauss Syndrome visit their healthcare provider?

The frequency of medical visits can vary depending on the severity of the condition and the phase of treatment. Initially, more frequent visits may be necessary to monitor the effectiveness of treatment and adjust medications. Once the condition is stable, visits may become less frequent but should still occur regularly to ensure ongoing management and early detection of any changes.

Can complementary therapies help manage Churg-Strauss Syndrome?

Some complementary therapies, such as acupuncture, massage, or herbal supplements, may provide relief for certain symptoms. However, it's important to discuss any complementary therapies with your healthcare provider before starting them, as they should not replace conventional treatments and may have interactions with prescribed medications.

References and Helpful Links

Amazon.com: Churg-Strauss Syndrome: A Beginner's Quick start guide on managing EGPA through home remedies and diet, with sample recipes eBook : Marshwell, Patrick : Kindle Store. (n.d.).
https://www.amazon.com/Churg-Strauss-Syndrome-Beginners-Managing-Remedies-ebook/dp/B0B4CXHSV2

Churg-Strauss Syndrome: A beginner's quick start guide on managing EGPA through home remedies and diet, with sample recipes. (2023, May 29). Everand.
https://www.everand.com/book/649298350/Churg-Strauss-Syndrome-A-Beginner-s-Quick-Start-Guide-on-Managing-EGPA-Through-Home-Remedies-and-Diet-With-Sample-Recipes

Eosinophilic Granulomatosis with Polyangiitis - Symptoms, Causes, Treatment | NORD. (n.d.). National Organization for Rare Disorders.
https://rarediseases.org/rare-diseases/churg-strauss-syndrome/

Churg-Strauss syndrome - Symptoms & causes - Mayo Clinic. (2024, February 7). Mayo Clinic.
https://www.mayoclinic.org/diseases-conditions/churg-strauss-syndrome/symptoms-causes/syc-20353760

Professional, C. C. M. (n.d.-c). EGPA (formerly Churg-Strauss Syndrome). Cleveland Clinic.
https://my.clevelandclinic.org/health/diseases/7098--eosinophilic-granulomatosis-with-polyangiitis-egpa-formerly-churg-strauss-syndrome

Yilmaz, I., Tutar, N., Simsek, Z. O., Oymak, F. S., & Gulmez, I. (2017). Clinical and Serological Features of Eosinophilic and Vasculitic Phases of Eosinophilic Granulomatosis with Poliangiitis: a Case Series of 15 Patients. Turkish Thoracic Journal, 18(3), 72–77. https://doi.org/10.5152/turkthoracj.2017.16040

Vasculitis UK. (2019, August 27). Diet and sensible eating for vasculitis patients - Vasculitis UK.
https://www.vasculitis.org.uk/living-with-vasculitis/diet

Asthma diet: Does what you eat make a difference? (2023, December 7). Mayo Clinic.
https://www.mayoclinic.org/diseases-conditions/asthma/expert-answers/asthma-diet/faq-20058105

www.ingramcontent.com/pod-product-compliance
Lightning Source LLC
LaVergne TN
LVHW012054070526
838201LV00083B/4579